Dyshidrotic Eczema (Pompholox):

Seeking Relief from the Itch and Blisters

By

Taylor Wyatt

Table of Contents

Acknowledgements

I thank God and my family for everything.

Introduction

All of a sudden, I had the unquenchable need to scratch the sides and tips of my fingers. The itchy areas began to have tiny little blisters and my skin hardened unlike anything I have ever seen before. My once perfectly manicured and baby doll- like hands began to resemble a science project. I was mortified. As my condition was misdiagnosed as simple dermatitis, I sought a second opinion and discovered that I had Dyshidrotic Eczema. Of course, this eczema is uncommon which makes coping more difficult.

As there is no known cure for this eczema, symptoms are generally treated with some form of oral or topical steroids. The long term effects of steroids (after consistent use) can be devastating. Therefore, I dedicate my current study of this condition to finding natural solutions to coping with Dyshidrotic Eczema as well as to help those suffering, understand this extremely annoying disease.

Part I.

Dyshidrotic Eczema

Some may find small vesicles or tiny blisters on their fingers. Although not contagious this form of eczema and the disfiguring tiny blisters (in some cases the blisters are large and painful) are simply unsightly. Again, there is no known cure for this type of eczema and even if skin clears the eczema can return, tiny blisters and all. According to the Mayo Clinic, Dyshidrotic Eczema usually appears or reappears during stressful situations, and annoying those with sensitive skin. It also becomes a problem for those coming in contact with certain metals such as chromium and nickel (2012). Furthermore, people suffering with atopic eczema are at risk for this type of eczema.

To simply sum up the question, *what is Dyshidrotic Eczema* (also known as pompholox), it is a form of eczema accompanied with blisters and severe itching and in some cases, painful blisters. There are no definitive reasons for this; however, there are theories that this type of eczema may be associated with an allergic reaction or for some, appear when allergies are most active.

I.   What are Common Treatments?

The use of topical corticosteroids is pretty common. Also, the use of UV light, and oral steroids have been prescribed in conventional medicine. Antihistamines are generally used to alleviate itching as well as the use of mineral oil and petroleum-based products. Minimizing hand washing and exposure to cleaning agents seems like a daunting challenge but is considered a solution.

Although there are a few items on the market than can help alleviate the discomforts associated with this form of eczema, maintaining daily duties and responsibilities is challenging. The use of corticosteroids may warrant more health trouble over time than the actual discomfort of itching. In using mineral oil and petroleum-based products, one will be promised a sure mess. Reducing the amount of hand washing is unfeasible, especially if your daily chores include diaper changing and cooking.

II.   The Roid and Side Effects

When first prescribed a topical corticosteroid, Triamcinolone Acetonide, I was elated. It seemed to stop the itching and within two to four days my skin seemed to improve. However, after many weeks of use, I noticed that I have been eating much more and have gained a significant amount of pounds. After steady use, the steroid seemed to have very little (if any) impact on my skin; the itching became more intense and I continued to be overwhelmed by frustration.

The use of steroids as a medical treatment has many benefits, but in some cases, the effects can be quite devastating. Of course, the strength of the prescription and how the medicine is being taken also impacts the degree of side effect. As noted by the Mayo Clinic, over time, inhaled steroids have the risk of fungal infections and hoarseness; topical steroids can contribute to acne, thin skin, and lesions; and oral corticosteroids can lead to increased eye pressure, impact mood, contribute to weight gain, and increased blood pressure (2012). Again, having a conversation with your physician is worth considering, especially with measuring the risks and the benefits of using steroids.

Part II.

Possible Scenarios worth Exploring

One of the most disheartening words for those suffering with Dyshidrotic Eczema is, *There is no cure for that*. Even at the beginning of this book I said the same thing. However, when these words are spoken by trusted members of the medical community, it destroys hope of breaking the vicious cycle of itching, scratching, cracking, and pain. In this section I will explore possible scenarios for flare-ups.

Scenario One: Stress as a Factor

Stress and stressful situations tend to incite a breakout, home remedies such as a cool compress and relaxing have been suggested but considering the intensity of itching and discomfort, the suggested home remedies are simply not powerful enough. Telling a miserably itchy person to *relax*, seems absurd. However, for many sufferers, including myself, flare-ups almost always occur in stressful situations and when stress is present.

As noted in an article by Koldys and Meyer, *Biofeedback training in the therapy of dyshidrosis*, biofeedback or the ability to control one's bodily functions has helped to alleviate flare-ups, particularly how the body reacts to stress (1979). I neither discredit nor agree with this, but I find it worth mentioning. In researching various articles and from personal experience, stress tends to incite flare-ups although it may not be the sole cause of this condition.

Scenario Two: Diet and Lifestyle as a Factor

Another suggested factor is diet and lifestyle. In finding causes of and cures for many diseases, diet and lifestyle can have a powerful impact on the human body. Many products sold in grocery stores, both edible and non edible contain some form of preservative or chemical to extend shelf life. Some soaps, body washes, dish detergents have chemicals as ingredients not only to extend shelf life, or to clean or whatever desired function, but also to give a product "color". Extending the discussion on coloring (including food coloring), food dyes such as Red 40 can be found in the most discreet places, such as in a can of biscuits or bubble bath!

Suffering from any medical condition warrants the need to read your labels and to be highly selective in what you purchase at stores. The same can also be translated to fast food products. The amount of chemicals used in fast food products is quite shocking and is worth considering as potential irritants just as the food dyes. Basically, if the product is processed, if human hands or machines manufactured the product, it is worth noting that it may be something you are ingesting or touching that makes you further susceptible to Dyshidrotic Eczema and other skin conditions. According to a study by Berglind, Alderling, & Meding, there is a strong probability that lifestyle (including diet and habits) impacts hand eczema:

> Hand eczema was more common in individuals who reported stress, obesity and smoking. In individuals who reported high physical exercise levels hand eczema was less common. As there appears to be an association between life-style factors and hand eczema it is important to consider life-style factors in
> clinical practice. (2011)

Such findings can bring to dialogue the possibility of controlling Dyshidrotic Eczema and other types of Eczema. In addition to the lack of exercise, popular preservatives and chemicals can also be considered as potential triggers. Considering their potential to incite flare-ups for the hypersensitive person, preservatives and chemicals can also have other ill impacts on your health. The subsequent chart highlights commonly used food preservatives, functions, sources and long term effects.

Beforehand, it is also fair to mention that some professions may make the already hypersensitive person more susceptible to this disease. Professions that require contact with metals and professions that require an excessive amount of handwashing can be the catalyst for Dyshidrosis.

Popular Preservatives

Name	Function	Sources	Side Effect
Red 40	Coloring	Gum, cereals, baked goods, soft drinks, juices, candy	Suspected to cause cancer, birth defects
BHT Butylated hydroxytoluene	Preservative	Various packaged foods	Behavioral Problems as hyperactivity; contribute to development of tumors and cancer
BHA Butylated hydroxyanisole	Preservative	Various packaged foods	Behavioral Problems as hyperactivity; contribute to development of tumors and cancer
Carmel Coloring	Thickener	Frozen pizza, artificially brown colored foods	Vitamin B6 deficiencies, certain cancers

Name	Function	Sources	Side Effect
Sodium Nitrate	Prevent fungal spoilage, prevent browning	Processed meats, packaged foods	Some forms of cancer
Benzoates	Preservatives	Fruit juices, margarine, tea and coffee extracts, flour, pickles	Brain damage, trigger allergies
Sulfur Dioxide	Bleaches food rot	Various packaged foods, including dried fruits and molasses	Toxin
Butylates	Preservative	Butter, margarine, vegetable oils	Elevated cholesterol levels, impairs liver and kidney functions
Refined Flour	Refined Foods	Junk foods, Fast foods	Elevates blood glucose levels, increase risk for obesity
Aspartame	Sweetener	Diet sodas, some sugar free products	Tumors, cancer

1 Ibrahim, S. (2010). Preserved Food hazardous. *Economic Review (05318955)*, *41*(3), 7.

Scenario Three: Metals as a Factor

According to Stuckert & Nedorost (2008) reducing the intake of Cobalt in the form of a low-cobalt diet may prove beneficial to alleviating flare-ups associated with Dyshidrotic Eczema. A different school of thought suggests hypersensitivity to nickel as a reason for hand eczema (Thyssen, 2011). Some researchers feel that certain metals can trigger this disease. In my research, Nickel has been deemed the more dominating culprit for this form of eczema than Colbalt. In an attempt to search for factors leading to Dyshidrotic Eczema, Lodi et al. (1992) conducted a study and reported roughly about 26% of the participants had traces of Nickel in their blood. Please note, the study does not determine Nickel as a cause of this eczema, but similar studies have also reported traces of Nickel in blood testing.

Nickel and Cobalt have been used in plating iron, brass, stainless steel, and in both silver and white gold (Thyssen, 2011). Consequently, prolonged exposure can lead to hypersensitivity or an allergy to Nickel and Cobalt and with exposure, dermatitis is quite likely to be present (Thyssen, 2011) which can make a case for the presence of Dyshidrotic Eczema. This revelation is not limited to the presence of these metals in jewelry; this can also be translated to those who work near or in an environment mostly consisting of exposure to these metals or those who frequently come in contact with such metals.

Again, evaluating lifestyle can provide insight regarding factors for flare-ups as well as answering any personal questions regarding Dyshidrotic Eczema. The food we consume, the objects we touch, and our place of work may secretly have an answer for why this form of eczema (or any other for that matter) exists.

Scenario Four: Predisposition

In one study, many of the dyshidrosis patients exhibited atopy or a susceptibility to allergens or factors to be attributed to allergens (Lodi, et al., 1992). This is translated to a hypersensitivity that makes certain people more susceptible to this disease than others. Some sufferers dealt with food allergies, environmental factors, and other allergy triggers. I can admit that

I suffer from food allergies and cannot consume food dyes or food powders (flavored drinks, powered cheese sauces) and based on this scenario, I can comprehend how atopy may play a role in Dyshidrosis.

Part III

Alternative Solutions to Dyshidrotic Eczema

If there is "no cure" for Dyshidrosis, in the medical community then finding alternative solutions should be the next proactive step to take in finding relief. In this section I explore some solutions to ease and hopefully diminish Dyshidrotic Eczema.

I. Exercise

Many studies find exercise as a method of reducing the chance of developing Dyshidrotic Eczema as well as quelling flare-ups in some people. Not only is exercise a stress reliever, but it also allows the body to rid of toxins. Additionally, exercise burns calories, which also helps reduce weight. Overall, exercise is a worthwhile venture to consider in fighting against many diseases, including Dyshidrotic Eczema. A little sweat can help. Walking, Jogging, and Pilates will afford rewarding workouts and Yoga is a great stress reliever as well as enhancing flexibility. Mixing and adding variations in your exercise routine will keep you engaged while adding benefits. Based on my personal experience, when I exercise consistently (three to four days a week for 45 minutes each session) my flare-ups are minimal, if there are any.

II.   Other Remedies

-Aloe vera juice or gel can reduce inflammation, heal cracked skin, and alleviate soreness. If you do not have fresh aloe vera (straight from the plant) purchase the unflavored, unsweetened juice from a drug store, get a small basin or container that affords enough room for you to place your hands (or the affected area), and soak the area for about twenty minutes as many times as you need. Even pouring a cup or two in your bath water can work while you soak. Remember, consistency is key and you must be consistent to see results.

-Synthetic UVA1treatments may be a suggested treatment for those with a more stubborn form of eczema. Considering synthetic UV treatments are used, some exposure to sunlight could prove beneficial in treating dyshidrotic eczema (Letic, 2009). Of course, do this with caution and discuss with your physician.

-It is documented that Evening Primose Oil can reduce inflammation and swelling as well as improve skin condition. The same is also noted of olive oil (Hoey, 2010). Both can be applied topically to the affected area or taken as supplements.

III.   Alkaline the Body

An acidic body can be a perfect host for diseases to thrive. Alkalizing the body will balance the ph levels of the body as well as to eliminate toxins. Although at this time there is not enough research to substantiate this claim, it is worth noting that positive dietary changes can assist in fighting against Dyshidrotic Eczema, which is what alkalizing the body professes. Moreover, alkalizing the body will help in losing weight! Remember, it is better to have a body that is alkaline than a body that is acidic.

The way to achieve an alkaline body is to reduce the intake of acidic foods and to increase the intake of alkaline foods. The following chart contains some examples of alkaline foods.

Alkaline Foods	Acidic Foods
Lemons, any other citrus, tomatoes, cucumber, carrots, lettuce, bananas, onions, apples, strawberries, peaches, apricot, and more	Any processed food, beans, meat, dairy products, almonds, rice, eggs, corn, and more

It is important to note that fresh, organic produce is best. If you are fortunate enough to have a produce stand in vicinity, locally grown produce is usually quite affordable and does not contain as much chemicals as produce sold in large conventional stores.

If you do not have the option of purchasing locally grown produce and buying organic produce is a bit too expensive, it is worthwhile to grow your own produce. Lettuce, carrots, herbs, tomatoes grow easily from seeds and with the right soil (organic and made for potting edible plants) these plants and others will continue to reward your efforts time and again. You can also purchase the plants, rather than the seeds from Home Depot and Lowe's. Any effort towards alkalizing your body can only help, especially once you minimize or eliminate processed foods and juices. **Un**processed food can only improve your overall health. Simply stated, if it's natural, there is a health benefit.

IV. Dead Sea Ingredients (*Nature's Beauty* brand)

Dead Sea ingredients have many healing benefits. The back story on this solution involves a trip I made to a flea market and meeting a vendor selling natural skin care products. The vendor works for a small, emerging company called **Nature's Beauty**. In trying the *True Dead Sea Mud*, I noticed that the uncontrollable, vicious itch stopped immediately once the mud was applied on my fingers. I even switched from conventional soaps, to washing my hands with *Nature's Beauty* Butter Soap. Since then, I became a firm believer and loyal customer of his. *Nature's Beauty* products are natural and do not use chemicals. With the permission of *Nature's Beauty*, I am able to include contact information in this book. You can visit their website at: www.naturesbeautyllc.com.

V.   Run From Sweets, Refined Carbs, and the Like

I cannot stress how important it is to consider the fact that refined and enriched foods, and I mean <u>everything</u> from cakes, pies, cookies, hot and cold breakfast cereal, biscuits, carbonated beverages, and even candies, can incite a flare-up. In fact, I took a challenge. I went two weeks without eating refined carbohydrates just to see if my skin will clear. And guess what, the itch was not there and my skin began to clear because I did not have the urge to scratch. This promoted healing! I maintained using the Butter Soap, being sure not to let chemicals and traditional soaps touch my skin, but in all honesty, I encourage you to take the two week challenge. You may even drop a couple pounds in the process while making your body alkaline!

Here is a sample meal plan:

Breakfast and Lunch:

A large salad (iceberg lettuce, romaine, carrots, red cabbage), ¼ cup shredded cheese, chopped chicken), carefully selected salad dressing, grapes (any fruit will do), Water or homemade Lemonade.

Dinner:

Any home cooked meal involving vegetables. My first favorite: Grilled Salmon or Chicken, steamed broccoli. My second favorite: Asian Stir fry. It is pretty similar to the first favorite meal except I add teriyaki and I stir fry the ingredients together. Water or homemade Lemonade is my beverage of choice.

Snacks:

I snack throughout the day. Fruit, Greek Yogurt (to get the "real" version consider purchasing from Whole Foods rather than buying the "filler" version. The "filler" version will have ingredients such as corn syrup, and additives for texture), and vegetables make a difference. There are times I really crave carbohydrates. For example, if I want a donut, I make my own using oatmeal flour and agave nectar as a sweetener. The bottom line, stay away from anything "enriched" or "refined". This fall you can find recipes or "substitutions" in my book, *Healthy and Sneaky, Substitutions.*

Conclusion

The intent of this book is to help fellow Dyshidrotic Eczema sufferers and others with similar skin conditions. In exploring what is Dyshidrotic Eczema, you already know the discomfort and anxiety associated with the condition. The book discussed conventional strategies as well as alternative, natural solutions. Also discussed in earnest were possible scenarios for explaining the condition.

Some people are hypersensitive to common objects and foods. Some may have to incorporate more exercise to fight off Dyshidrosis and the mere fact that stress is a factor in many diseases is quite aligned with the scenario of stress being a factor in this condition. As a person that has been diagnosed with this condition, the mere conclusion, *there is no cure for that"* is simply unacceptable.

The contents of this book is not to discredit the medical community but rather to extend research and time as well as providing personal experience in order to help others. I hope you have gained more clarification and hope in fighting this condition. Remember, you are not alone in this.

References

Berglind, I., Alderling, M., & Meding, B. (2011). Life-style factors and hand eczema. *The British Journal Of Dermatology, 165*(3), 568-575. doi:10.1111/j.1365-2133.2011.10394.x

Hoey, N. (2010). Natural Dyshidrosis Eczema Cures. Livestrong.

Ibrahim, S. (2010). Preserved Food hazardous. *Economic Review (05318955), 41*(3), 7.

Koldys, K., & Meyer, R. (1979). Biofeedback training in the therapy of dyshidrosis. *Cutis; Cutaneous Medicine For The Practitioner, 24*(2), 219-221.

Letić, M. (2009). Exposure to sunlight as adjuvant therapy for dyshidrotic eczema. *Medical Hypotheses, 73*(2), 203-204. doi:10.1016/j.mehy.2008.08.035

Lodi, A., Betti, R., Chiarelli, G., Urbani, C., & Crosti, C. (1992). Epidemiological, clinical and allergological observations on pompholyx. *Contact Dermatitis, 26*(1), 17-21.

Mayo Clinic. (2012). Dyshidrosis: Risk Factors. Retrieved from: http://www.mayoclinic.com/health/dyshidrosis/DS00804/DSECTION=risk-factors

Nature's Beauty, LLC. (2013).
WWW.Naturesbeautyllc.com.
info@naturesbeautyll.com.

Stuckert, J., & Nedorost, S. (2008). Low-cobalt diet
for dyshidrotic eczema patients. *Contact
Dermatitis, 59*(6), 361-365. doi:10.1111/j.1600-
0536.2008.01469.x

Thyssen, J. (2011). Nickel and cobalt allergy
before and after nickel regulation--evaluation of
a public health intervention. *Contact Dermatitis,
65 Suppl 1*1-68. doi:10.1111/j.1600-
0536.2011.01957.x

The information provided in this book does not substitute the advice and care of a physician.

www.ingramcontent.com/pod-product-compliance
Lightning Source LLC
Chambersburg PA
CBHW030548290526
45786CB00004B/1926